CONGRATULATIONS ON YOUR DECISION TO GET HEALTHY!

The 21 Day Salad Fast
(Healthily Eat Your Way Thin)

COOKBOOK III

A guide to a *new eating plan* that is not a "DIET", created based on personal experience to help you *finally* achieve your weight loss and health goals.

ALSO BY KYLA LATRICE, MBA

"New Me, New You! (How I Overcame Obesity)"

"The 7 Day Smoothie Detox"

"The 21 Day Slushie & Juice Fast"

"The 21 Day Salad Fast"

"Eat Well and Stay Thin (Living a Healthy You)"

"21 Days to a New Healthy You! Hearty Vegan & Vegetarian Slow Cooker Recipes"

"Twenty-One Healthy Ice Pop Snack Recipes"

"21 Days of Everyday Healthy Snack Recipes"

"All Natural Soups & Stews"

"A Collection of My Favorite Health Recipes"

"A New You! Workout Workbook"

THE 21 DAY SALAD FAST
Healthily Eat Your Way Thin

A 21 DAY SALAD FAST TO RESET YOUR HEALTH, MIND, BODY, METABOLISM AND *"LIFE"*

KYLA LATRICE, MBA

Lady Mirage Publications, Inc.

New York   Memphis   Los Angeles   London   Cape Town   Toronto
Atlanta   Singapore   Japan

Copyright © 2014 by Ms. Kyla Latrice, Inc.
The author is represented by Lady Mirage Literary Agency, Inc.
All rights reserved. In accordance with the U.S. Copyright Act of 1976, the scanning, uploading, and electronic sharing of any part of this book without the permission of the publisher is unlawful piracy and theft of the author's intellectual property. If you would like to use material from the book (other than for review purposes), prior written permission must be obtained by contacting the publisher at
www.LadyMirageAgency.com
Thank you for your support of the author's rights.

Published by:
Lady Mirage Publications, Inc.
3724 Goodman Rd W, Unit 575
Horn Lake, MS 38637
www.LadyMirageAgency.com

Manufactured in the United States of America
First Edition: July 2014

Lady Mirage Publications, Inc. is an imprint and subsidiary of Lady Mirage Global. The Lady Mirage Publications, Inc. name and logo are trademarks of Lady Mirage Global.

Authors within the Lady Mirage Global (under Lady Mirage Agency, Inc.), Lady Mirage Publications and Lady Mirage Literary Agency speakers division provides a wide range of authors for speaking engagements. To find out more information, go to
www.LadyMirageAgency.com
Cover photo provided by Derek Murphy at CreativeIndie

The publisher is not responsible for websites (or their content) that are not owned by the publisher.

Library of Congress Cataloging-in-Publication Data:
eISBN: 978-1-31-111101-2; Print ISBN: 978-0-9975371-0-9
Tennin, Kyla Latrice.
The 21 Day Salad Fast
Pages cm; copyrighted materials.
1. Health-Nutrition-Diet-Fitness. 2. Cooking. 3. Fitness.
Library of Congress Catalog Card Number: 2016907243

Print Book Edition, License Note

This book is licensed for your personal enjoyment only. This book may not be re-sold or given away to other people. If you would like to share this book with another person, please purchase an additional copy for each recipient.
If you're reading this book and did not purchase it, or it was not purchased for your use only, then please return to your favorite book retailer and purchase your own copy. Thank you for respecting the hard work of this author.

Also Note

In this book, Ms. Latrice begins by explaining a *fast* that she has created, tested and tried, which contributed to her weight loss, weight management and healthy eating lifestyle journey. She has also written this book due to there being so many books, health, weight-loss and "diet" programs currently on the global market. The programs and books she has seen and reviewed are too long, too thick, have too much information and many times, are difficult for people to read. This book was written to ***simplify and shorten*** how to lose weight and maintain your health, for life. It is based on personal experience and is still done today. It's an effective solution.

The 21 Day Salad Fast
(Healthily Eat Your Way Thin)

Table of Contents

GREEN-SALAD RECIPES..40
- Day 1: Dried Tomato Basil Traditional…...…............42
  - Day 2: Garlic Chicken...………………..…......................44
- Day 3: Red Bell Pepper Delight……………...............46
  - Day 4: Quinoa Salad with Pears…......................…...48
- Day 5: Pineapple Salad with Sesame Dressing……….50
  - Day 6: Avocado Dill Salad……………...........................52
- Day 7: Sesame Cider Vinegar Salad…………...…........54
  - Day 8: Pineapple Dill Remix……………...................56
- Day 9: Macadamia Nut Salad…………….…...............58
  - Day 10: Salmon Carrot Lime Salad………….........60
- Day 11: Blueberry Coconut Salad…………….............62
  - Day 12: Quinoa Pesto Salad……………...................…..64
- Day 13: Dried Oregano Feta Salad……………...........66
  - Day 14: Summer Kiwi Salad……………….............…..68
- Day 15: Kyla's Vegan Cobb Salad………………..........70
  - Day 16: Tilapia Fajita Salad……………....….………...72
- Day 17: Strawberry Pecan Salad…………….............74
  - Day 18: Cucumber Feta Salad with Balsamic…….76
- Day 19: Cashew Chicken Mango Salad…………...…...78
  - Day 20: Shrimp Avocado Salad……………...............82
- Day 21: Vegan Taco Salad……………….…..….................80

INDEX……………..….....84
- Green-Salad Recipes…………….....…………….84

DEDICATION

This cookbook is dedicated to men and women around the world that have dealt with or are beginning to deal with food addiction, obesity and/or declining health.

I also dedicate this book to those whom have been "Mirage's" in life; overlooked, betrayed, not good enough, slandered, mistreated, misunderstood, misrepresented and even treated unfairly because of their weight or how they looked on the *outside* to others, when in fact, on the *inside* there's greater.

This new cookbook is also dedicated to men and women around the world that want to
shift from being ordinary to extraordinary and accomplishing what others said you would never be able to do again or never be able to do at all.

Here's to the New You!

ACKNOWLEDGMENTS

I want to *say thank you* to anyone whom has ever betrayed,
rejected, mistreated, teased, and misused
or looked down upon me. You helped me become GREATER
and launched me into my destiny.

Whenever someone throws bricks at you, use them to *"build"*.
Build something greater; even your mansion.

And whenever you face opposition, "know" that it is actually
an opportunity; a set-back for a set-up to secure the victory,
rejection for rewards, pain for gain, lack for prosperity to
leave a legacy, misery for miracles and put downs for
promotion.

IT'S YOUR TIME…*to bounce back!*

Let's Get Healthy!

AUTHOR'S NOTE

The 21 Day Salad Fast (Healthily Eat Your Way Thin)
Copyright © 2014
Ms. Kyla Latrice, Inc.
All Rights Reserved.

AFFIDAVIT

All content written herein is of opinion, from personal experience and of suggestion. Individual salad fast and new eating plan results may vary from person to person and no results are guaranteed.

You must put forth effort and do the work necessary to take charge of changing your life and *losing weight*. I did and so can you.

You can also utilize this cookbook if you have already met your weight loss goals and just want to stay healthy with recipes that will keep your metabolism in check and body running smoothly.

Be sure to wash all fruits, vegetables, foods, etc. thoroughly before beginning any new
eating or meal plan.

ALL RIGHTS RESERVED

No portion of this publication may be reproduced, stored in any electronic system, or transmitted in any form by any means; electronic, mechanical,
photocopy, recording or otherwise, without written permission from the author.

Brief quotations may be used in literary reviews with the consent of the author and publisher.

THE 21 DAY SALAD FAST | HEALTHILY EAT YOUR WAY THIN

"ON-THE-GO"

This cookbook *(and all of my cookbooks, books, workbook and manuals)* can be read and applied in airports, on trains, at work on your lunch break, in grocery stores while shopping for and planning your weekly meals, at bookstore cafes, at restaurants *(for quick decision making; to remember your health and/or weight loss goals)* and even in shopping malls.

In addition, *this book can be brought to* fast food restaurants (to pull up and look through to remember your goals before ordering), at the park (before a jog or potluck), during your hotel stays, on vacations and at airport food counters when ordering your meals and drinks *(so you remember your goals and what to eat and drink)*.

This cookbook has been made available on mobile devices via Adobe Digital Editions and DRM (Digital Rights Management).

WORLD STATISTICS

Obesity and Childhood Obesity
Centers for Disease Control and Prevention
http://www.cdc.gov/obesity/data/adult.html
http://www.cdc.gov/nchs/fastats/obesity-overweight.htm

Harvard School of Public Health
http://www.hsph.harvard.edu/obesity-prevention-source/obesity-trends/

World Health Organization
http://www.who.int/topics/obesity/en/

Stroke Awareness and Prevention
http://www.cdc.gov/stroke/facts.htm

Diabetes Awareness and Prevention
Centers for Disease Control and Prevention
http://www.cdc.gov/diabetes/data/statistics/2014statisticsreport.html

American Diabetes Association
http://www.diabetes.org/diabetes-basics/statistics/

"FASTING"

WHAT IS FASTING?
- Fasting is abstaining from PLEASURABLE foods for a certain amount of time to FOCUS on things that are more important than pleasurable foods to get to the root of what is causing your poor health, obesity, relationships and quality of life.

- It is not a hunger strike.

- You're able to see into your life better and rid it of the bad when you pull away from portion after portion at the dinner table, lunch buffet after buffet with friends and co-workers, nightly binge eating and drinking (whether alcohol, sodas, sugary drinks and the like) and dessert or movie nights on the sofa with a large pizza box and donuts.

- Fasting helps you pinpoint where you overdo things (overindulge), gets you back on track and teaches you how to eat, "in moderation" (balance), for your health and for a better life.

- Your body may not like eating healthy for the first few days (especially if you have never fasted before), but it will adjust.

REASONS FOR FASTING:
- It produces a physical discipline (especially for how, when, where and *what* you eat).

- It rids the body of toxins (just like exercise does when you sweat); cleansing your body and digestive tracts, improving your health and weight.

Note: If you are on medication, consult your physician before any *fast*.

BENEFITS OF FASTING:
- It strengthens *you* and your body.

- Fasting brings joy, happiness and *energy* to your life; and fruits, vegetables, oils, etc. are quite inexpensive. Make a list and shop for your ingredients before you begin.

- You become very aware of *what* and *how much* you eat. You also begin to pay more attention to when and where you always eat/drink and what leads you to OVEREATING.

- Fasting brings humility, revelation and an overall healthy lifestyle (mind, emotions, intellect, etc.).

TYPICAL TYPES OF FASTS:
Sometimes people fast the following from their lives:
- Television (even the internet, social media or video games) for one day, three days or even one week, television during certain hours of the day (to break a cycle of watching certain shows they may be addicted to (like food) that aren't good for them.

    ....or
- To break a cycle of "certain foods" they may eat while watching certain television shows.

- Fasting to abstain from all pleasurable foods and red meats, eating only fruits, vegetables, clear soups, cereals (no white sugar), water, diluted fruit juices (100% juices only) and/or grains.

- Some people even fast people (bad acquaintances, friendships or relationships), leading eventually to moving away from those person's completely, for a better life and health. Your health is your life.

- Many people fast for 24 hours, three days, seven days, 14 days, 21 days or longer. My success and learning my body as well as other persons bodies (whom have fasted when I have fasted) has come from "closely monitoring" how the body reacts to each of these fasts (particularly "21 days") and I've noticed some things and have sculpted recipes to help others find that tremendous success in many areas of their lives as well.

- Fasts should always be broken slowly, especially if you have been on an "extended fast" (a fast for more than 30 days, a salad only fast, a smoothie only fast or even a clear soup only fast).

- Gradually get back into "regular food", until you can completely commit to "healthy food" (and a regular healthy lifestyle); such as having juices for a couple of days, then fruits, vegetables, grains and adding meats back into your diet last, if applicable.

- Typically, people have six meals per day (three main meals (breakfast, lunch and dinner) and three snacks). For each of my Fasts or Recipes, you determine how many meals. Don't worry, fruits and vegetables do not cause obesity, they prevent it. Yet, always watch your portion sizes, in general, and with soups, stews and anything that has meat included. Never eat meat in excess.

- You can even choose to eat one meal per day for 21 days (there are enough recipes listed in this book), a snack, have 5-8 bottles of water and be sure to get a nap in and some exercise during the week. As you advance you can mix your salad fast with a smoothie fast and detox fast by doing one of the fasts, each per week, for 21 days, etc.

THE *"SALAD FAST"* BIRTH

Kyla Latrice is a native of Marks, MS and enjoys food and traveling. Being from a small town and a country gal, she set her goals high. Graduating from a private institution with a Bachelor of Arts Degree (BA) *(women's studies and health background; pre-medicine)* and a Master's Degree (MBA) in Business Administration with **Executive Education at Harvard and Stanford** along with several certifications and nearly 50-80 self-study coursework in legal, intellectual property and self-help, she has become one of the leading entrepreneurs of her time.

Currently Ms. Latrice is finishing up her Doctoral Honorary Degree *(Doctor of Management in Organizational Leadership)* and continues to serve on Board of Directors throughout the world for various causes; still relating to her life's purpose and corporations work. Ms. Latrice travels extensively for speaking engagements in the areas of health, wellness, obesity, poverty, domestic violence, branding, image, leadership, mentoring, business, entrepreneurship and the like.

To date, Ms. Latrice has mentored with over 20 plus organizations *(from elementary to senior citizen)*, helping others overcome issues she has faced.

With her first *corporate* job opportunity being at a "Health Food Restaurant" *(when she was age 15 or 16)* to work as a deli attendant at the deli bar, hostess *(when others were out for the day)* and bakery attendant as well as a chef in the *salad bar*.

Her main role was to attend to the deli, to prepare healthy pasta salads, healthy sandwiches, healthy shakes, healthy sundaes and *healthy smoothies*. However, Ms. Latrice was blessed with the opportunity to be called upon whenever management needed her help in the other areas as well, **to continue learning**. This gave Ms. Latrice very valuable experience and a "look" into health and business ownership, a bit deeper, which still remains with her today.

THE *"SALAD FAST"* BIRTH

KYLA LATRICE
BEFORE
21 DAY SALAD FASTS

Ms. Latrice's *(on the left in the photo)* Corporations are inclusive of health restaurants, retail stores, property and land as well as product development organizations along with nonprofit foundations to care for the displaced, homeless.

Further, Ms. Latrice's love for food turned into obesity when her life took a turn in the early 2000's during domestic violence, sinful relationships, bad friendships and emotional binge eating; then again in the 2000's with another domestic violence relationship, obesity slander from family members, mental and spiritual abuse, abortion, home foreclosure, vehicle repossession and much *more*, which all have an effect on health, but she made sure her Corporations still stood; to help others.

THE *"SALAD FAST"* BIRTH

KYLA LATRICE
"IN THE MIDDLE"
AFTER GAINING WEIGHT BACK FOR A SECOND TIME
21 DAY SALAD FASTS

THE *"SALAD FAST"* BIRTH

KYLA LATRICE
AFTER
21 DAY SALAD FASTS

THE FINALE

Many factors can contribute to obesity, such as abuse *(mental, spiritual, physical, sexual)*, poor eating habits, environment, bad friendships as well as sin. Personally, I, myself, was never taught how to eat, I did not know what to eat *(that was truly healthy for me)* and I did not know how to deal with life's problems.

Nevertheless, how can someone teach you what they don't know? My first encounter with obesity was when I was a model and went from a size 0 to a size 20/22, **weighing close to 300 pounds** *(then I lost nearly 115 pounds after prayer and seeking a remedy)*.

The second encounter was when I gained some of the first encounters weight back and went from a size 14/16 to a size 4/6 and fitting a 7/8 in jeans, losing 68 pounds. Today, I am going to share my secrets to success with you *(the birth of the "21 Day Salad Fast")* and how I made it out over the years ***and*** kept the weight off. Let's get started and healthy, for life!

GETTING HEALTHY
LIFESTYLE CHANGE

THE 21 DAY SALAD FAST | HEALTHILY EAT YOUR WAY THIN

Prepare to lose weight on the "Salad Fast" (this is not a "diet", this is an "eating plan" to reprogram your mind, body and metabolism about how to eat (portion control) and regarding what foods you should and should not be eating). It is designed to help you become healthier. Before starting this fast and any of my eating *plans ("The 21 Day Smoothie Fast" and "The 21 Day Salad Fast" as well as "Soups and Stews")*, allow yourself "one week" to prepare for the fast and eating plan by removing the following from your life:

➢ Negative relationships and friendships; they block you from doing well in life and succeeding, when people begin to see you doing well, they tend to not like it. Choose friendships and associations wisely. Be creative.

➢ Bad acquaintances; they will eventually want what you have and will cause betrayal to take place in your life through a "set-up" to sabotage all of your hard work. Always keep moving forward.

➢ Remove the following (slowly) from your daily meals (eating habits) because they contribute to weight gain (some quicker than others): soda, breads, pastas, candy bars and the like and eating second, third and fourth portions of your food. You only need one portion. Don't eat the rest!

➢ Replace all sodas with diet soda until you can cut soda out of your daily meal plan completely; only drink soda if absolutely necessary *(a lemon-lime beverage)* because there is nothing else to drink. For example, while traveling.

➢ Remove all "junk food" (cakes, pies, chips, all kinds of desserts and the like) from your kitchen.

- For breads, certain kinds make the weight gain skyrocket; be careful about pizza. Pasta should be limited just like soda, having it only if absolutely necessary, but once every 2-4 months is okay, just like donuts, to stay **balanced** and give your body a break from always eating healthy.

- Again, you only need one portion of food, per meal, work on this and you'll see results quicker.

- Increase your water intake to 5-8 bottled waters a day; bring a bottle with you everywhere you go so you'll be forced to drink it *(instead of something else)* and will program your body to like it *(whether you like it frozen, warm or cold)*.

- When you're out to eating with others, begin selecting items from menus that help *(not hinder)* your **new eating plan**, for example, order a "grilled chicken wrap with a side salad and small water" instead of a double cheeseburger, french fries and large soda. Never super-size, it wastes your results and time spent on improving your health.

- If you have not already, purchase my books: *"The 21 Day Smoothie Fast"* and *"The 7 Day Detox"* to begin, to continue your weight loss and new you.

- And again, remember, commit to single portion eating, eating smaller portions (always have more vegetables on your plate than poultry/ meat), and increase your water intake *(remember to use the restroom)*. Let's begin.

GETTING HEALTHY
SET GOALS

Feel free to purchase my "A New Healthy You Workout Workbook" *(to go with your **new eating plan** and my "fasts" cookbooks* or a composition notebook from any retailer to make your own journal to measure the following (even if you need to do so at your primary care physician's office, a free clinic or go to a free health assessment machine in a retail store location that has one):

Record a written record of each:

- Your Cholesterol Level.
- Blood Pressure and Vision Check.
- Your actual Height Weight, Height, Bust/Chest and Hips size (write down your goals of where you want to be in the next week, three months, six months and year).
- Record your weight, chest/bust, hips and waist size every Saturday morning at 7am.
- Stroll through a department store and notate clothing (or take a camera phone photo) you plan on fitting into someday and notate your current sizes and then return in three months to see how you're fairing up towards your goals.
- Pick up my *"A New Healthy You Workout Workbook"* or list in your journal, your reasons for losing weight, changing your life and changing your eating habits.

- Your BMI (Body Mass Index) and where you are versus where you're supposed to be for your height, weight, age and gender.
- Bottles of "cold water" listed in the recipes section of this book are in reference to drinking 4-5 bottles of 16 fl oz bottles of water, which is equivalent to 8-10 glasses of water per day.
- Water is vital for living and for being healthy.
- The amount of water within the human body is typically 50-65% water and in infants, 78%.
- Water assists your body with digesting food and getting nutrients from the foods you have eaten to your blood, brain and other parts of your body, in order to function; emptying the body of waste and toxins, helps deliver oxygen to the body, helps prevent constipation and even regulates body temperature (in your cells, organs and tissues).

A (BMI) Chart is below for your convenience.

BMI	<(less than) 18.5	=	Underweight
BMI	18.5-24.9	=	Normal Weight
BMI	25-29.9	=	Overweight
BMI	>(more than) 30	=	Obese

GETTING HEALTHY
WHILE TRAVELING

If you'll be traveling by airplane, helicopter or private jet (smile):

- ➢ Research where you will be eating ahead of time (food choices, ingredients and prices).
- ➢ Bring bottled water.
- ➢ Resist vending machines and relying of fast food at your final destination.
- ➢ Bring your own snacks (trail mix, cashews, a banana, apple slices, peanuts) and
- ➢ Workout for free in your hotel room, taking the stairs instead of elevators and walking at the Mall.

If traveling by car:

- ➢ Pack your own cooler with ice for your bottled waters, fruits and raw vegetables.
- ➢ Consider bringing a bag of oranges & any other food that can be eaten warm or cold on the road.

If you'll be traveling by bus, train, or other means:

- ➢ Research where you will be eating ahead of time (food choices, ingredients and prices).
- ➢ Bring bottled water.
- ➢ Bring your own snacks (trail mix, cashews, a banana, apple slices, peanuts for the long trip) and
- ➢ Bring something to read or play, to keep your mind off of food and *fictious* hunger.
- ➢ At your destination, stand more than you sit (to keep your body moving) and since you have been sitting during traveling for your trip.

ASPARAGUS

Photo Credit: SOMMAI
FREEDIGITALPHOTOS.NET

GETTING HEALTHY
YOUR NEW WORKOUT PLAN

During my both times of being obese, I never worked out at a gym nor went outside of my home to run *(weighing in at 278 pounds and trying to start my "new me" as a jogger was terrible on my knees)* to lose weight, I did it all at home, on the floor, in a compact room, near a closet. I suggest you begin a "workout regime" by doing simple workouts, such as crunches, stretching, leg lifts and a few push-ups.

Everyone cannot do cardio in the gym (paid membership prices or because of lack of transportation), running outside or bouncing around in-doors for 1-3 hours like actors and actresses on television, whom are likely being *paid monetary* compensation or by other means to film the infomercial.

Remain constant and do this 3-4 times a week, for 15-35 minutes each day. On your workout OFF days, do 100 crunches before going to bed. Consider purchasing my "Workout Workbook" to keep up with your Fitness Plan. In addition, you burn calories when you sleep, by drinking water, by exercising (which helps you live longer as well) and by **movement** (whether your arms, legs, looking out of a window, etc.).

Furthermore, water helps break down food and helps food digest. Your can also do a "mental workout" by cutting out negative people, places and things from your life.

You'll find that you have more peace in your brain and life, when you replace them with reading inspirational books, movies, community work and exercise or things you love, such as knitting, a ball game, taking a site seeing road trip (alone) every now and then or mentoring someone.

Notes

THE SIX MONTH RULE
GIVE IT *"TIME"*

THE SIX-MONTH RULE
On a 21-Day Salad Fast, weight [pounds] have been known to drop quickly for many people. However, the goal here is to also keep the weight off. Stay focused and be committed to at least six-months of "health work".

Remember to journal your progress.

There's something about when you write things down, they get *ACCOMPLISHED!* Also give yourself a total of six-months to work on your "New You" simply because you may lose inches first and not weight, until your weight catches up with your inches (this is what took place with me; loosing 10-12 pounds per month).

Inches first then one day the weight just fell off. And for others, sometimes weight first, then inches.

GO BACK TO THE DEPARTMENT STORE
Revisit those same department stores that you went to on the first week of your new lifestyle change, try on new clothing sizes to see where you are with your goals.

I suggest that you "mentally shop" for a new suit, a dinner dress, clothing for you next vacation (Hawaii maybe), your first pair of skinny jeans or baseball gear to wear to a game; all after you have reached your goals; to *CELEBRATE!*

"GREEN-SALAD" RECIPES

WEEK 1
ARUGULA WEEK

Photo Credit: Apolonia
FREEDIGITALPHOTOS.NET

WEEK 1, DAY 1
(DRIED TOMATO BASIL TRADITIONAL)

Day 1 of Week 1: Dried Basil, Extra-Virgin Olive Oil, Fresh Lemon Juice, Shredded Skinless Boneless Rotisserie Chicken Breast, Diced Roma Tomatoes

Add 1/2 teaspoon of dried basil into a large salad bowl, Add 3 tablespoons of extra-virgin olive oil, Add 1/2 of a lemon's squeezed juice, Add 1 cup of shredded skinless boneless rotisserie chicken breast, 1/2 cup of diced Roma Tomatoes, Mix salad with large serving spoon until evenly mixed, Place on a bed of baby arugula on a dinner plate or in a to go container, Serve immediately

Health Notes:

Dried Basil – Basil is great for cooking, making pesto as well as for relieving coughs, colds, infections, high blood sugar levels, stress and headaches. These leaves are also great for calming the stomach, soothing it from indigestion and feeling too full (in general and from overeating) due to their many nutrients, including but not limited to Vitamins K, A, C and Iron, Folate, Magnesium as well as Copper.

Extra-Virgin Olive Oil– Extra-Virgin Olive Oil is rich in Omega 6 and Omega 3 as well as Vitamin's E and K. Olive oil can also be found in Avocados, Nuts and Fatty Fish. This olive oil also has antioxidants that have the ability to heal a body's internal cells, protecting the outer later from damage (skin, nails and eyes).

Weight Loss Tip: Drink 4-5 bottles of cold water today.

GARLIC

Photo Credit: Suat Eman
FREEDIGITALPHOTOS.NET

WEEK 1, DAY 2
(GARLIC CHICKEN)

Day 2 of Week 1: Garlic, Extra-Virgin Olive Oil, Fresh Lemon Juice, Shredded Skinless Boneless Rotisserie Chicken Breast, Green Onions

Add 1/2 teaspoon of minced garlic into a large salad bowl, Add 3 tablespoons of extra-virgin olive oil, Add 1/2 of a lemon's squeezed juice, Add 1 cup of shredded skinless boneless rotisserie chicken breast, 1/2 cup of diced green onions, Mix salad with large serving spoon until evenly mixed, Place on a bed of baby arugula on a dinner plate or in a to go container, Serve immediately

Health Notes:

Garlic – Garlic is an excellent source of nutrient that promotes overall body health. It relaxes blood vessels and increases blood flow, reducing heart disease. In addition, garlic boosts the immune system, prevents athlete's foot (fungus on the feet), hair loss *(with its ancillian properties)*, clears acne from the skin, helps reduce weight, helps heal cold sores, inflammation, food poisoning (like E. coli and Salmonella) and hypertension and cancers.

Green Onions– Green Onions help boost your nutrition and are rich in vitamins, minerals and phytochemicals, helping with your overall bone health (Vitamins K and C; which are crucial for the growth, development and maintenance of strong bones to reduce bone fractures as well as osteoporosis), eye health (Vitamin A), immune health (DNA and cellular tissues) and heart health (Vitamin C) to reduce risk of heart disease.

Weight Loss Tip: Drink 4-5 bottles of cold water today.

THE 21 DAY SALAD FAST | HEALTHILY EAT YOUR WAY THIN

GREEN BEANS

Photo Credit: SOMMAI
FREEDIGITALPHOTOS.NET

WEEK 1, DAY 3
(RED BELL PEPPER DELIGHT)

Day 3 of Week 1: Red Bell Peppers, Extra-Virgin Olive Oil, Fresh Lemon Juice, Shredded Baked Lemon Chicken Breast, Green Beans

Add 1 cup of a diced red bell pepper into a large salad bowl, Add 1 cup of green beans, Add 3 tablespoons of extra-virgin olive oil, Add 1 Lemon Chicken Breast, Add 1/2 of a lemon's squeezed juice, Mix salad with large serving spoon until evenly mixed, Place on a bed of baby arugula on a dinner plate or in a to go container, Serve immediately

Health Notes:

Red Bell Pepper – These bell peppers are great when roasted or eaten raw. They are rich in Vitamins C, E and B6 aiding in lowering bad cholesterol and pain from inflammation. Red Bell Peppers also help keep your skin and hair looking youthful (Vitamin K) and prevent certain cancers. They are also low in calories and help maintain weight while also helping to protect the eyes from cataracts and macular degeneration and help renew cells in the nervous system (Vitamin E).

Green Beans– Fresh Green Beans (not canned) are great for your health. They're rich in Vitamins C & A, Manganese, Folates and Fiber as well as low in calories making them great for snacks, salads and healthy meals. Green Beans also help treat acne, prevent aging and aid in hair care.

Lemon Juice – Lemons are a great source of citric acid, Vitamins C, Calcium and even Potassium. They also help fight hair loss, lumps on the skin and hands, high blood pressure, arthritis, constipation, vision loss, excess gas, gallstones, internal bleeding, fevers and indigestion and aids in cleansing the teeth & dandruff from the hair.

Weight Loss Tip: Drink 4-5 bottles of cold water today.

PARSLEY

Photo Credit: James Baker
FREEDIGITALPHOTOS.NET

WEEK1, DAY 4
(QUINOA SALAD WITH PEARS)

Day 4 of Week 1: Almonds, Extra-Virgin Olive Oil, Chopped Parsley, Quinoa, Pears

    Add 1 cup of a diced almonds into a large salad bowl, Add 2 cups of diced pears, Add 1 cup of chopped parsley, Add 1 cup of rinsed and cooked quinoa, Add 2 tablespoons of extra-virgin olive oil, Mix salad with large serving spoon until evenly mixed, Place on a bed of baby arugula on a dinner plate or in a to go container, Serve immediately

Health Notes:

Almonds – Almonds are an interesting nut. They help reduce heart attack risk, lower blood sugar, bad cholesterol, build strong bones and teeth due to their Phosphorus content, protect artery walls from damage (with their Flavonoids and Vitamin E), nourish the nervous system and the healthy fats in almonds also aid in weight loss. They also prevent certain cancers, inflammation and are known to improve skin condition.

Quinoa– Quinoa (gluten free and low in calories) is a seed that comes from a vegetable related to spinach and beets and is high in protein and even has more protein compared to some rice and wheat. Quinoa also helps promote healthy skin, energy metabolism in the brain and muscle cells, also aiding in weight loss and weight management due to its low glycemic index. It also needs washing before cooking or eating.

Arugula – Arugula is rich in Vitamins A, C and K and promotes cellular reproduction, eye health, immunity boosting, helping poor vision, improves respiratory and skin health, cleanses and detoxifies the body, helps clean out the colon and helps with bowel movements, fights cancers, boosts oxygen levels, body repair (building tissue), prevents blood clots and protects against birth defects.

Weight Loss Tip: Drink 4-5 bottles of cold water today.

AVOCADO

Photo Credit: Master Isolated Images
FREEDIGITALPHOTOS.NET

WEEK 1, DAY 5
(PINEAPPLE SALAD WITH SESAME DRESSING)

Day 5 of Week 1: Pineapple, Honey, Ginger with Sesame Oil, Avocado, Egg

Add 1 cup of a diced chilled pineapple into a large salad bowl, Add 3 diced hard-boiled eggs, Add 2 tablespoons of sesame oil with a tablespoon of ginger chopped and mixed in, Add 2 tablespoons of honey, Add 1 whole diced avocado, Mix salad with large serving spoon until evenly mixed, Place on a bed of baby arugula on a dinner plate or in a to go container, Serve immediately

Health Notes:

Avocado – Avocado are rich in Vitamins E, C and monounsaturated fats, aiding in Arthritis and Diabetes prevention, helping a heart stay healthy and reducing the risk of cardiovascular disease. They also aid in weight loss and clearing skin (signs of aging) due to their Vitamins C & E and antioxidant content. Avocados also have disease fighting compounds in them, like beta-carotene and lutein. They are also rich in Potassium (more than bananas have) and aid in promoting overall body health.

Honey– Honey really does come from bees, from their nectar and is rich in Fructose, Glucose, Sucrose, Maltose, Water, Iron, Calcium, Phosphate, Magnesium *(a mineral and nutrient that helps you relax, maintain energy level and helps sustain the health of your heart and blood vessels as well as alleviate constipation and prevents heart attacks and strokes)* and even Sodium Chloride. Honey helps with coughs and colds, is an anti-bacterial and anti-fungal, helps prevent cancers, ulcers, gastrointestinal disorders and heart disease and aids in repairing chronic wounds.

Weight Loss Tip: Drink 4-5 bottles of cold water today.

WALNUTS

Photo Credit: Suat Eman
FREEDITIALPHOTOS.NET

WEEK 1, DAY 6
(AVOCADO DILL SALAD)

Day 6 of Week 1: Walnuts, Avocado, Cilantro, Grilled Chicken Strips, Fresh Dill

Add 1 cup of a walnuts into a large salad bowl, Add 1 whole diced avocado, Add 1/2 cup of cilantro, Add 1 cup of fresh dill, Add 2-3 chopped grilled chicken strips, Mix salad with large serving spoon until evenly mixed, Place on a bed of baby arugula on a dinner plate or in a to go container, Serve immediately

Health Notes:

Walnuts – Raw nuts such as Almonds, Cashews and Walnuts have been linked to lower cholesterol, are a great snack (especially when mixed together), aid in bettering your overall health, preventing cancer risk and lowering and controlling weight. Walnuts also help protect the body from cell damage that contributes to heart disease, inflammation, are rich in Vitamin E (helping lower bad cholesterol and weight gain) and are rich in Zinc to help deliver oxygen to the body's cells and prevent anemia.

Cilantro– Most people use Cilantro (similar to "dill") in wraps, salads, pastas, pesto, guacamole and even soups. However, really, it can be used in anything. Cilantro is rich in Magnesium, Iron and antioxidants, helping the body fight aging, chronic diseases and food poisoning *(Salmonella; bacteria)*. Due to Cilantros anti-microbial properties and phytonutrients it also helps aid in curing yeast infections, kidney stones and sleep disorders.

Weight Loss Tip: Drink 4-5 bottles of cold water today.

(BLACK) SESAME SEED

Photo Credit: Naypong
FREEDIGITALPHOTOS.NET

WEEK 1, DAY 7
(SESAME CIDER VINEGAR SALAD)

Day 7 of Week 1: Sesame seeds, Almonds, Cranberries, Cucumbers, Cider Vinegar

Add 1 cup of a diced almonds into a large salad bowl, Add 2 cups of sesame seeds, Add ½ of a diced cucumber, Add 1 cup of diced cranberries, Add 2 tablespoons of cider vinegar, Mix salad with large serving spoon until evenly mixed, Place on a bed of baby arugula on a dinner plate or in a to go container, Serve immediately

Health Notes:

Sesame Seed – Sesame seeds contain B Vitamins, Calcium, Iron, Manganese, Copper, Magnesium, Fiber, Zinc, Vitamin B6, Protein, Phosphorous as well as Thiamin. The Vitamins and Minerals in Sesame Seeds / Sesame Seed Oil is great for oral health, preventing diabetes, reducing blood pressure, boosts digestive health and prevents Asthma (due to their magnesium content; preventing airway spasms). They also detoxify the body, iron deficiency, kidney damage and possibly even multiple sclerosis (MS).

Cranberries– Cranberries are high in fiber and Vitamin C, helping the kidneys and to prevent urinary tract infections (UTIs). They also have no fat and no sodium making them a favorite for those with bladder problems. Cranberries also help fight tooth decay. Cranberry Juice flushes out your system and speeds up weight loss with antioxidants.

Cider Vinegar– Cider vinegar also helps detoxify your body, improve your skin health (the skin's pH, when applied as a moisturizer), removes stains from teeth, aid in weight loss when mixed with water (due to its Triglycerides fighting content), improves digestion, bad breath, acne, kidney stones, hair loss, and menopause and strengthens the immune system.

Weight Loss Tip: Drink 4-5 bottles of cold water today.

WEEK 2
MIXED ROMAINE & RED CABBAGE WEEK

Photo Credit: SOMMAI
FREEDIGITALPHOTOS.NET

WEEK 2, DAY 8
(PINEAPPLE DILL REMIX)

Day 1 of Week 2: Pineapple, Green Bell Pepper, Salt/Pepper, Lemon Juice, Dill

Add 1 cup of a diced pineapple into a large salad bowl, Add 1 cup of chopped green bell pepper, Add a dash of salt and pepper to season, Add 1/2 of a squeezed lemons juice, Add 1 cup of freshly chopped dill, Mix salad with large serving spoon until evenly mixed, Place on a bed of mixed romaine with 1/2 cup of a chopped red cabbage mixed in on a dinner plate or in a to go container, Serve immediately

Health Notes:

Dill– Dill contains anti-oxidant disease preventing properties and are rich in Vitamins A, C, Potassium, Copper, B2 (Riboflavin) as well as Zinc and beta-carotene. Dill helps with insomnia, bone health, hiccups, digestion, diarrhea and with removing excess water, gas, salt and toxins from the body. Dill also helps regulate menstrual cycles (menstrual cramps); prevents genital ulcers, infections, bronchitis and even fevers, liver and gallbladder issues (urinary tract infections).

Romaine– Rich in Omega 3's, Iron, Vitamin C (more than oranges have), Water as well as Calcium and protein, this plant also has a great source of Vitamin K. Romaine is good for your bones, teeth, eye health, night vision, impaired color vision and fighting allergies.

Red Cabbage – Red Cabbage is low in calories and fat and high in fiber and Vitamin K, making it ideal for weight loss, mental function and concentration. It also helps detoxify the body (helping to preventing arthritis, rheumatism, gout and even skin diseases), lower blood pressure and even blood sugar. Its Vitamin C content protects cells from damage and strengthen the body's muscles and tissues.

Weight Loss Tip: Drink 4-5 bottles of cold water today.

DILL

Photo Credit: James Barker
FREEDITIALPHOTOS.NET

WEEK 2, DAY 9
(MACADAMIA NUT SALAD)

Day 2 of Week 2: Poppy Seed, Dill, Honey, Ginseng, Macadamia Nut Oil

Add 1 cup of poppy seeds into a large salad bowl, Add 1 cup of freshly chopped dill, Add 2 tablespoons of honey, add a small portion of ginseng, Add 1/2 cup of macadamia nut oil, Mix salad with large serving spoon until evenly mixed, Place on a bed of mixed romaine with 1/2 cup of a chopped red cabbage mixed in on a dinner plate or in a to go container, Serve immediately

Health Notes:

Poppy Seeds– Poppy seeds contain niacin and folate as well as Calcium, Phosphorus (to build bones and prevent osteoporosis) Iron and Zinc (aids in neurological development and prevents immune system deficiencies). They also aid in digestion and preventing heart, digestive and stomach disorders as well as insomnia, diarrhea, asthmas and even whopping cough.

Ginseng– Ginseng comes in Asian, Korean or American. Ginseng helps improve mood and helps fight fatigue, cancers, heart disease, hepatitis C, menopausal systems and high blood sugar levels. Ginseng also boosts energy, concentration and learning. It also helps slow the signs of aging, reduces stress and menstrual cramps, aids in weight loss (fighting obesity) and fights diabetes.

Macadamia Nut Oil – This oil is rich in dietary fiber and is gluten free. Macadamia Nuts also help reduce bad cholesterol in the body and high blood pressure.

Weight Loss Tip: Drink 4-5 bottles of cold water today.

APPLES

Photo Credit: Paul
FREEDIGITALPHOTOS.NET

WEEK 2, DAY 10
(SALMON CARROT LIME SALAD)

Day 3 of Week 2: Apple, Carrot, Lime Salmon, Fresh Thyme, Salt/Pepper

Add 2 diced green apples into a large salad bowl, Add 1 diced carrot, Add 1 chopped (already prepared baked piece of salmon with a limes juice cooked in), Add fresh thyme, season with a dash of salt and pepper, Mix salad with large serving spoon until evenly mixed, Place on a bed of mixed romaine with 1/2 cup of a chopped red cabbage mixed in on a dinner plate or in a to go container, Serve immediately

Health Notes:

Apples– Apples help whiten your teeth by producing saliva, assisting with reducing tooth decay, protects against cancers, gallstones, hemorrhoids, constipation and high cholesterol. They also help you control your weight, prevent cataracts, decrease your chances of developing diabetes and boost your immune system (red apples; which have an antioxidant called quercetin in them). Apples are also packed with Vitamins C, A and Flavonoids, Phosphorus, Iron and Calcium as well as Potassium to help promote heart health.

Limes – Limes are rich in Vitamin C and folate. Interestingly, you may think, the juice, fruit and peel of a lime are used to make medicines and help cure severe diarrhea. Limes also kill germs in the skin, aiding in skin care *(preventing aging);* they ease constipation and help prevent fever, urinary tract and bladder infections, ulcers, heart disease *(lowering bad cholesterol)* and even arthritis.

Thyme – Thyme helps cure colds (with its antiseptic and antibiotic properties) and improves vision because of its rich Vitamin A content and antioxidant properties promoting healthy vision.

Weight Loss Tip: Drink 4-5 bottles of cold water today.

BLUEBERRIES

Photo Credit: Ambro
FREEDITIGALPHOTOS.NET

WEEK 2, DAY 11
(BLUEBERRY COCONUT SALAD)

Day 4 of Week 2: Blueberries, Raspberries, Lemon, Salmon, Coconut Oil

Add 1 cup of blueberries into a salad bowl, Add 1 cup of raspberries, Add 1/2 of a lemon (diced), Add 1 tablespoon of coconut oil, Add 1 chopped (already prepared baked piece of salmon), Mix salad with large serving spoon until evenly mixed, Place on a bed of mixed romaine's with 1/2 cup of a chopped red cabbage mixed in on a dinner plate or in a to go container, Serve immediately

Health Notes:

Blueberries– Blueberries are infused with great sources of Vitamins C and E, riboflavin, niacin and folate. Blueberries also have proanthocyanidins (to help fight aging) and phytonutrients ellagic acid (anticancer protection) in them along with catechins *to help burn abdominal fat to double weight loss.*

Salmon – Salmon aid in overall heart, brain and nerve health. Salmon also help lower your risk of developing Alzheimer's and Parkinson disease.

Coconut Oil – Coconut Oil has a great effect on health and is rich in fatty acids that fight obesity. Coconut Oil increases energy, kills bacteria, fungi and even some viruses aiding in warding off infections. The oil is also rich in Lauric Acid which assists with killing the pathogens of bacteria, fungi and viruses associated with disease. Coconut Oil also helps skin heal faster, treats athlete's foot, psoriasis and eczema and is also used for bathing, deodorant and hair care. It also helps with mental alertness, allergies and can be used to deep fry food.

Weight Loss Tip: Drink 4-5 bottles of cold water today.

ASPARAGUS

Photo Credit: SOMMAI
FREEDIGITALPHOTOS.NET

WEEK 2, DAY 12
(QUINOA PESTO SALAD)

Day 5 of Week 2: Quinoa, Pesto, Balsamic Vinegar, Roma Tomatoes, Asparagus

Add 1/2 cup of rinsed and cooked quinoa into a salad bowl, Add 2 teaspoons of pesto, Add 1 tablespoon of Balsamic Vinegar, Add 1 cup of diced roma tomatoes, Add 2-3 diced stalks of asparagus, Mix salad with large serving spoon until evenly mixed, Place on a bed of mixed romaine with 1/2 cup of a chopped red cabbage mixed in on a dinner plate or in a to go container, Serve immediately

Health Notes:

Pesto – Pesto sauce is made from olive oil, parmesan cheese, pine nuts, fresh basil and garlic *(all put into a blender to make a sauce)*. Pesto is rich in Vitamins A and C, promoting strong bones, healthy red blood cells, building tissue in the body, supporting eye health and fights disease causing free radicals in the body.

Balsamic Vinegar – Vinegar slows digestion and makes you feel fuller sooner, preventing overeating leading to weight gain and severe obesity. Balsamic Vinegar is also naturally sweetened, decreasing the need for sugar and/or additional sugar in your food or drinks. Balsamic Vinegar is also rich in antioxidants aiding in reducing cholesterol. It also helps reduce unhealthy fats and sodium in the body.

Asparagus – Asparagus contains detoxifying properties, Vitamins K, B (to help regulate blood sugar levels) A (for better vision), C, E, Iron and Inulin (a prebiotic that supports the "good" bacteria in our guts). Asparagus is also rich in fiber, low in starch and helps lower high blood pressure and heart related issues.

Weight Loss Tip: Drink 4-5 bottles of cold water today.

OREGANO

Photo Credit: James Barker
FREEDIGITALPHOTOS.NET

WEEK 2, DAY 13
(DRIED OREGANO FETA SALAD)

Day 6 of Week 2: Carrot, Tomato, Dried Oregano, Cucumber and Feta Cheese

Add 1 diced carrot into a salad bowl, Add 1/2 cup of diced roma tomatoes, Add 1 teaspoon of dried oregano, Add 1 cup of crumbled feta, Add ½ of a diced cucumber, Add 2 tablespoons of 100% extra virgin olive-oil, Mix salad with large serving spoon until evenly mixed, Place on a bed of mixed romaine with 1/2 cup of a chopped red cabbage mixed in on a dinner plate or in a to go container, Serve immediately

Health Notes:

Oregano – Oregano is rich in Vitamins K & E, Iron, minerals, Fiber and Omega-3 fatty acids which all help in promoting overall body health, fighting acne, dandruff and even bone issues (helping to maintain bone density and preventing blood clots). Oregano also includes antioxidants to help fight infections.

Feta – Feta cheese is a cheese that is made with sheep or goat's milk and has a semi-hard texture. Feta cheese is rich in protein and low in calories, making it ideal for pastas and salads, aiding in low daily calorie intake and **weight management.**

Carrots – Carrots can be white, yellow, red, purple and orange. They are also great for your teeth, killing off harmful germs in the mouth to help prevent tooth decay. Carrots also have a great source of Vitamin A, beta carotene *(an antioxidant to help maintain healthy skin),* Alkaline elements (which help purify and revitalize the blood) and Potassium *(helping the body maintain normal blood pressure levels).*

Weight Loss Tip: Drink 4-5 bottles of cold water today.

KIWI

Photo Credit: SOMMAI
FREEDIGITALPHOTOS.NET

WEEK 2, DAY 14
(SUMMER KIWI SALAD)

Day 7 of Week 2: Kiwi, Pineapple, Nectarines, Walnuts, Honey

Add 1 cup of a diced kiwi into a salad bowl, Add 1 cup of diced pineapple, Add 1/2 cup of diced nectarines, Add 1 cup of walnuts, Add 2 tablespoons of Honey, Mix salad with large serving spoon until evenly mixed, Place on a bed of mixed romaine with 1/2 cup of a chopped red cabbage mixed in on a dinner plate or in a to go container, Serve immediately

Health Notes:

Nectarines – Nectarines are a low calorie fruit rich in dietary fiber, Magnesium, Folate, Potassium, Vitamins A, E, C, B6, B4 (Niacin), B2 (Riboflavin), B1 (Thiamine), K, beta-carotene and Luetin (aiding in eye health), to name a few (nutrients). They also contain Chlorogenic acid which fights obesity related conditions like diabetes and cardiac issues; heart disease and bad (high) cholesterol. They also aid in digestion, cellular health and preventing hypokalemia (muscular degeneration).

Kiwi – Kiwi fruit is a small powerhouse that helps manage blood pressure because of its high level of potassium and helps with digestion. Kiwi is high in fiber and low glycemic index for weight loss, rich in immunity booster Vitamin C and carries Vitamin E for clearer skin; also fighting heart disease and cleaning toxins from the body.

Walnuts – Walnuts are an antioxidant that has an anti-inflammatory benefit which aids in preventing cardiovascular problems, cancers, type 2 diabetes (a chronic disease where there are high levels of glucose/sugar in the blood) as well as metabolic syndrome (a cluster of biochemical and physiological abnormalities that are related to type 2 diabetes).

Weight Loss Tip: Drink 4-5 bottles of cold water today.

WEEK 3
SPINACH WEEK

Photo Credit: Smarnd
FREEDIGITALPHOTOS.NET

WEEK 3, DAY 15
(KYLA'S VEGAN COBB SALAD)

Day 1 of Week 3: Avocado, Kidney Beans, Cherry Tomatoes, Boiled Egg, Green Onion

      Add 1 cup of cooked kidney beans into a salad bowl, Add 1 cup of diced cherry tomatoes, Add 2-3 diced hard boiled eggs, Add 2-3 stalks of diced green onion, Add 1 whole diced avocado, Mix salad with large serving spoon until evenly mixed, Place on a bed of spinach on a dinner plate or in a to go container, Serve immediately

Health Notes:

Kidney Beans – These beans are full of nutrients, mineral, folate and proteins, low in calories and sodium and help reduce cancers and **organ damage**. They are also rich in Vitamins A, C, Iron, Potassium and Magnesium; promoting a stronger cardiovascular system.

Cherry Tomatoes – Cherry tomatoes are rich in Vitamin A and also contain high amounts of Chromium to help maintain blood sugar levels in the body. They also contain Potassium and Vitamin B to help lower cholesterol and blood pressure. Cherry Tomatoes are about the same size as a cherry and are most of the time sweeter and juicer than other tomatoes. Tomatoes in general reduce heart disease, prevent DNA damage, protect against Thrombosis (blood clots in blood vessels), cancers and inflammation.

(Boiled) Egg – Boiled eggs are rich in B12 and Vitamin A. The nutrients within boiled eggs help support strong bones, eye health, reproduction, teeth and skin. They are also low in calories, contain Vitamin E, folate, iron and zinc and are great on salads, aiding in **weight management**.

Weight Loss Tip: Drink 4-5 bottles of cold water today.

THE 21 DAY SALAD FAST | HEALTHILY EAT YOUR WAY THIN

LIMES

Photo Credit: Master Isolated Images
FREEDITIALPHOTOS.NET

WEEK 3, DAY 16
(TALAPIA FAJITA SALAD)

Day 2 of Week 3: Tilapia, Bowtie, Ginger, Lime, Dried Oregano

Add 1 cup of cooked (whole grain wheat) bowtie pasta into a salad bowl, Add 2 whole baked and diced tilapia, Add 1 knob of fresh ginger (small portion), Add the zest of 1 lime and the limes juice, Add 1 teaspoon of dried oregano, Mix salad with large serving spoon until evenly mixed, Place on a bed of spinach on a dinner plate or in a to go container, Serve immediately

Health Notes:

Lime – Limes are rich in Vitamin C and folate. Interestingly, you may think, the juice, fruit and peel of a lime are used to make medicines and help cure severe diarrhea. Limes also kill germs in the skin, aiding in skin care *(preventing aging);* they ease constipation and help prevent fever, urinary tract and bladder infections, ulcers, heart disease *(lowering bad cholesterol)* and even arthritis.

Oregano – Oregano is rich in Vitamins K & E, Iron, minerals, Fiber and Omega-3 fatty acids which all help in promoting overall body health, fighting acne, dandruff and even bone issues (helping to maintain bone density and preventing blood clots). Oregano also includes antioxidants to help fight infections.

Weight Loss Tip: Drink 4-5 bottles of cold water today.

STRAWBERRIES

Photo Credit: Ambro
FREEDIGITALPHOTOS.NET

WEEK 3, DAY 17
(STRAWBERRY PECAN SALAD)

Day 3 of Week 3: Spinach, Pecans, Grape Seed Oil, Goat Cheese, Strawberries

Add 1/2 cup of diced spinach into a salad bowl, Add 1 cup of pecans, Add 2 tablespoons of grape-seed oil, Add 2 ounces of fresh goat cheese, Add 2 cups of diced strawberries, Mix salad with large serving spoon until evenly mixed, Place on a bed of spinach on a dinner plate or in a to go container, Serve immediately

Health Notes:

Strawberries – Strawberries improve blood sugar regulation and are high in fiber and help BURN stored fat. They are packed with antioxidants (like Vitamin C) to help fight wrinkles and ease Inflammation. They also contain Vitamin K, potassium and magnesium. Nitrate is also included in these sweethearts for weight loss.

Grape Seed Oil – Grape Seed Oil is good for your hair (preventing moisture loss) and skin and helps regulate blood circulation. It also tones skin, helps fight heart disease and helps with acne, asthma and arthritis swelling. It is odorless, light and can also be used as a hot oil treatment. It is also among the three [most] healthiest oils: Grape-seed, Avocado Oil and Walnut Oil. Grape-seed oil is also rich in Vitamin E and polyunsaturated fats, aiding in boosting good cholesterol in the body, lowering bad cholesterol and fighting the development of diabetes.

Goat Cheese – Goat cheese is rich in Calcium, Vitamins A & K, Thiamin, Niacin and even Phosphorus. Fats found in goat milk are easier for the body to process than cow's milk, promoting an overall healthy diet (body).

Weight Loss Tip: Drink 4-5 bottles of cold water today.

CUCUMBERS

Photo Credit: SOMMAI
FREEDIGITALPHOTOS.NET

WEEK 3, DAY 18
(CUCUMBER FETA SALAD WITH BALSAMIC)

Day 4 of Week 3: Cherry Tomatoes, Black Olives, Feta Cheese, Cucumbers, Balsamic Vinegar

Add 1 cup of a diced cherry tomatoes into a salad bowl, Add 1 cup of diced black olives, Add an ounce of feta cheese, Add 1 cup of a diced cucumber, Add 1 tablespoon of balsamic vinegar to season, Mix salad with large serving spoon until evenly mixed with (whole grain wheat) bowtie pasta, Place on a dinner plate or in a to go container, Serve immediately (can also be served cold, the next day)

Health Notes:

Feta Cheese – Feta cheese is a cheese that is made with sheep or goat's milk and has a semi-hard texture. Feta cheese is rich protein and low in calories, making it ideal for pastas and salads, aiding in low daily calorie intake and **weight management.**

Cucumbers – Cucumbers are in the family of melons, squash and pumpkins. They are a great source of Vitamins K, C, A and B and are made up 95% water and are great for the eyes, skin and hair due to their anti-inflammatory properties and hair growth stimulation. They also help fight cancers (ovarian, uterine, breast as well as prostate) and aid in **weight loss**, digestion, blood pressure control, cholesterol reduction and joint pain relief (that is associated with arthritis). Cucumbers also dissolve kidney stones and rid the body of waste products.

Goat Cheese – Goat cheese is rich in Calcium, Vitamins A & K, Thiamin, Niacin and even Phosphorus. Fats found in goat milk are easier for the body to process than cow's milk, promoting an overall healthy diet (body).

Weight Loss Tip: Drink 4-5 bottles of cold water today.

THE 21 DAY SALAD FAST | HEALTHILY EAT YOUR WAY THIN

MANGOS

Photo Credit: SOMMAI
FREEDIGITALPHOTOS.NET

WEEK 3, DAY 19
(CASHEW CHICKEN MANGO SALAD)

Day 5 of Week 3: Avocado, Grilled Chicken Breast Chunks, Mango, Cashews, Lemon Juice

Add 1 diced grilled chicken breast into a salad bowl, Add 1 whole diced mango, Add 1/2 cup of cashews, Add 1/2 of an avocado diced, Add 1 whole lemons juice, Mix salad with large serving spoon until evenly mixed, Place on a bed of spinach on a dinner plate or in a to go container, Serve immediately (can also be served cold, the next day)

Health Notes:

Mangoes – Mangoes are rich in Vitamins A (antioxidant and vision) and C (antioxidant and immune booster) as well as Vitamins B6, copper, potassium, beta-carotene, magnesium and even healthy probiotic fiber. Mangoes also help clear skin (acne and clogged pores), fight cancer, lower cholesterol, help digestion, aids in weight loss, and aids in memory health and are high in iron for women.

Avocado – Avocado are rich in Vitamins E, C and monounsaturated fats, aiding in Arthritis and Diabetes prevention, helping your heart stay healthy and reducing the risk of cardiovascular disease. They also aid in weight loss and clearing skin (signs of aging) due to their Vitamins C & E and antioxidant content. Avocados also have disease fighting compounds in them, like beta-carotene and Lutein. They are also rich in Potassium (more than bananas have) and aid in promoting overall body health.

Weight Loss Tip: Drink 4-5 bottles of cold water today.

AVOCADOS

Photo Credit: MASTER ISOLATED IMAGES
FREEDIGITALPHOTOS.NET

WEEK 3, DAY 20
(SHRIMP AVOCADO SALAD)

Day 6 of Week 3: Black Pepper, Avocado, Shrimp, Cilantro, Sesame Oil

Add 1 cup of a whole diced avocado into a salad bowl, Add 1/2 cup of cilantro, Add 2 tablespoons of sesame oil, Add a dash of black pepper and sea salt to season, Add 2 cups of diced (cooked; baked or sautéed in butter) shrimp (tail removed) Mix salad with large serving spoon until evenly mixed, Place on a bed of spinach on a dinner plate or in a to go container, Serve immediately

Health Notes:

(Black) Pepper – Black pepper (a spice and a medicine) is beneficial the less its heated and helps improve digestion and promote overall intestinal health; I love it on my cobb salads and soups as well as in my tuna salad and on my custom made egg salad *sandwiches (the pepper helps with weight loss by breaking down fat cells)*. Black pepper is also high in dietary fiber, B Vitamins (B1, B2, B3, B6, B12 and even Biotin (for hair, skin and nail health) & Folate), A Vitamins D and E, including mineral proteins and low in calories. This pepper also comes in white. Black pepper helps with relief from respiratory disorder, coughs, indigestion, anemia, dental diseases, constipation and even diarrhea.

Sesame Oil - Sesame seeds contain B Vitamins, Calcium, Iron, Manganese, Copper, Magnesium, Fiber, Zinc, Vitamins B6, Protein, Phosphorous as well as Thiamin. The Vitamins and Minerals in Sesame Seeds / Sesame Seed Oil is great for oral health (reducing the amount of streptococcus mutants in teeth plaque and mouth saliva), preventing diabetes, reducing blood pressure, preventing DNA damage and cancers. They also detoxify the body and prevent iron deficiency.

Weight Loss Tip: Drink 4-5 bottles of cold water today.

CILANTRO

Photo Credit: SOMMAI
FREEDIGITALPHOTOS.NET

WEEK 3, DAY 21
(VEGAN TACO SALAD)

Day 7 of Week 3: Cherry Tomatoes, Cilantro, Avocado, Cheddar Cheese, Corn

Add 1/2 cup of a diced cherry tomatoes into a salad bowl, Add 1/2 cup of a diced Avocado, Add 1/2 cup of grated sharp white cheddar cheese, Add ½ cup of diced cilantro, Add 3 ears of corn (kernels cut off), Add 1/2 cup of 100% Extra Virgin Olive Oil, Mix salad with large serving spoon until evenly mixed, Place on a bed of spinach on a dinner plate or in a to go container, Serve immediately

Health Notes:

Cherry Tomatoes – Cherry tomatoes are rich in Vitamin A and also contain high amounts of Chromium to help maintain blood sugar levels in the body. They also contain Potassium and Vitamin B to help lower cholesterol and high blood pressure. Cherry Tomatoes are about the same size as a cherry and are most of the time sweeter and juicer than other tomatoes. Tomatoes in general help reduce heart disease, prevent DNA damage, protect against Thrombosis (blood clots in blood vessels), cancers and inflammation.

Spinach – Spinach are filled with Vitamins C, E, beta-carotene and even zinc. They also have a large amount of Vitamin K *(helping with brain function)* helping the nervous system and fighting stroke and cardiovascular disease. They also help maintain strong bones and prevent excess activation of osteoclasts (cells that break down bones). Spinach also help prevent osteoporosis, high blood pressure, vision *problems (protecting the eyes from cataracts and macular degeneration as you age)* and immune deficiencies *(such as urinary, respiratory and intestinal tract infections; strengthening these tracts).*

Weight Loss Tip: Drink 4-5 bottles of cold water today.

CONGRATULATIONS ON YOUR NEW YOU!

*Keep up the great work by continuing
on with my two newest books, "The 21 Day Smoothie Fast"
and the "The 7 Day Detox"*

INDEX OF RECIPES

DAY 1	42	DAY 12	64
DAY 2	44	DAY 13	66
DAY 3	46	DAY 14	68
DAY 4	48	DAY 15	70
DAY 5	50	DAY 16	72
DAY 6	52	DAY 17	74
DAY 7	54	DAY 18	76
DAY 8	56	DAY 19	78
DAY 9	58	DAY 20	80
DAY 10	60	DAY 21	82
DAY 11	62		

www.ingramcontent.com/pod-product-compliance
Lightning Source LLC
Chambersburg PA
CBHW071841090426
42811CB00035B/2303/J